Potty Training

Your step by step guide for little boys and little girls

Elizabeth Paterson

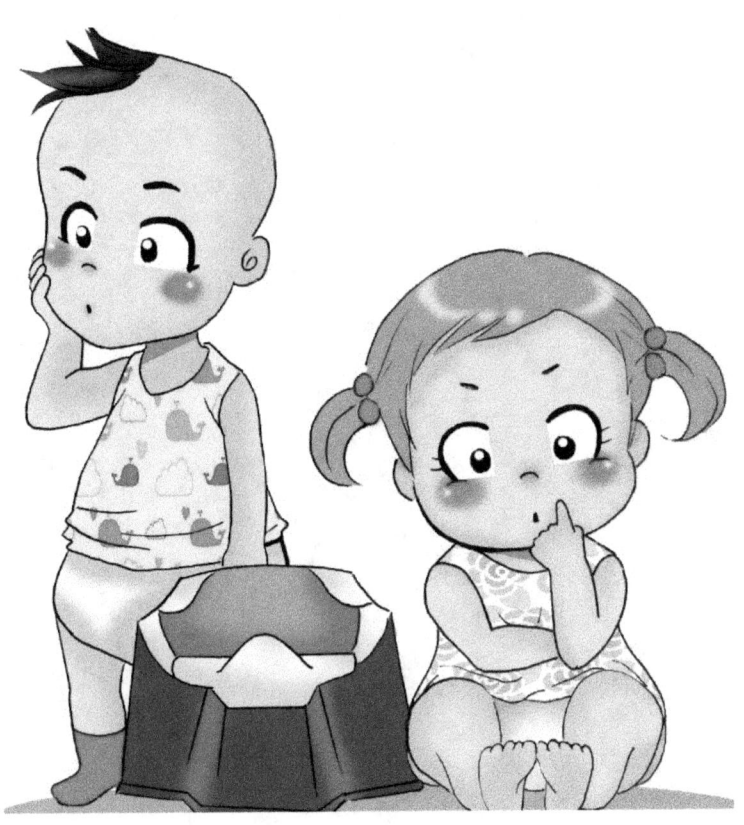

© Copyright 2018 by Beryl Assets LLC - All rights reserved worldwide.

This document is geared towards providing exact and reliable information regarding the topic and issue covered. The publication is sold with the idea that the publisher is not required to render accounting, officially permitted, or otherwise, qualified services. If advice is necessary, legal or professional, a practiced individual in the profession should be ordered.

- From a Declaration of Principles which was accepted and approved equally by a Committee of the American Bar Association and a Committee of Publishers and Associations.

In no way is it legal to reproduce, duplicate, or transmit any part of this document in either electronic means or in printed format. Recording of this publication is strictly prohibited and any storage of this document is not allowed unless with written permission from the publisher. All rights reserved.

The information provided herein is stated to be truthful and consistent, in that any liability, in terms of inattention or otherwise, by any usage or abuse of any policies, processes, or directions contained within is the solitary and utter responsibility of the recipient reader. Under no circumstances will any legal responsibility or blame be held against the publisher for any reparation, damages, or monetary loss due to the information herein, either directly or indirectly.

Respective authors own all copyrights not held by the publisher.

The information herein is offered for informational purposes solely and is universal as so. The presentation of the information is without contract or any type of guarantee assurance. The reader should understand that this book is not a substitute for competent medical advice and that the author is not engaged in the business of rendering any medical advice.

The trademarks that are used are without any consent, and the publication of the trademark is without permission or backing by the trademark owner. All trademarks and brands within this book are for clarifying purposes only and are the owned by the owners themselves, not affiliated with this document.

Table of Contents

Here We Are! It's Potty Training Time!	1
Some Simple Medical Facts	7
Classic Parents' Mistakes	11
The Readiness of The Child	19
How Do Parents Go About Training Children?	27
Main Potty-Training Methods	31
Problems Faced by Parents	41
Medical Problems	57
When Should the Parents Seek Help?	61
Children with Special Needs	65
Some Final Tips	69
Conclusion	73
References	75

Here We Are! It's Potty-Training Time!

Potty training usually begins between the ages of 18 months and 3 years. Some kids are early, and for some others it comes a little later, so to speak. Potty training is an important milestone in your child's early development helping to establish independence and self-confidence. It marks the transition between being a little baby and being a little boy or a little girl. It is also an exciting moment for the parents, after all you won't have to deal with dirty (and expensive) diapers anymore. At the same time, it is often a dreaded moment. I am sure that the thought of an accident has already crossed your mind more than once! Accidents are part of the process and they will likely happen, but there are ways to anticipate them and to reduce the risks. As a matter of fact, parents are often pressured by family members and teachers at the daycare, sometimes even by friends and co-workers, who may or may not even have kids themselves. I have been there, two times. In fact, it seems that, when it comes to your kid's education and well-being, everybody has an opinion about what, when and how you should do things. And Potty training is no exception. If some opinions may be helpful, there is also a lot of misinformation and unnecessary pressure on the parents.

In this book I will provide you with *all* the relevant information that you may need during this process.

Potty-training a child is neither rocket science nor does it have to be a long and protracted process. Several training methods exist. If it is possible to train your child in just a day or two, most methods will help you reach this result in less than a week, provided your child is ready for it. Every child is different, and I want to reassure you if it takes longer for your child or if you keep hearing that your child should already be potty trained not to worry.

For now, what you should keep in mind is that:

- Potty training is a natural milestone (with a little push from the parents);

- All children are not alike. What works for one may not work for another, and some kids will learn faster than others. This is just the way it is;

- There may be occasions when a child will need the help of an expert;

- Except in very rare cases, even children with special needs *do* succeed in potty-training;

- In any case, patience and perseverance pay off, with

pleasant results for parents and children all around.

Some Simple Medical Facts

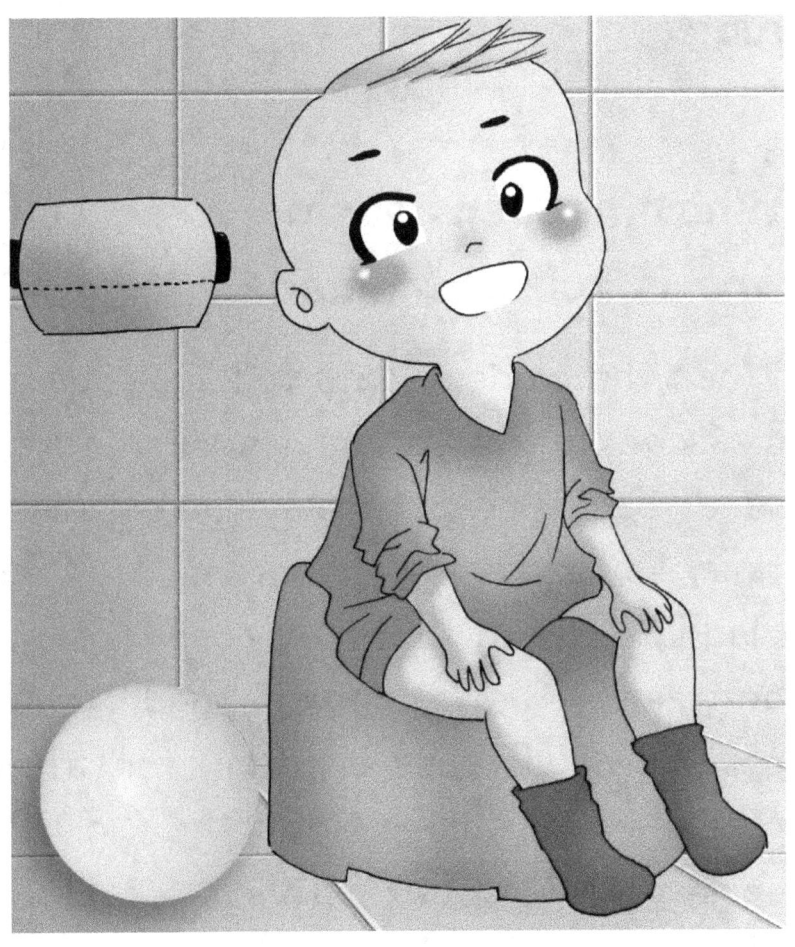

Let's start with some basic medical facts that will help you understand in layman terms what happens inside our bodies and what differentiates adults and young children with respect to our subject.

What happens inside a person who is toilet-trained:

When the bladder gets full, it sends a message to the brain, which in turn sends back a response saying that it is time to empty the content of the bladder. Hence, it takes coordination between the central and the peripheral nervous system for the proper functioning of the lower urinary tract. Emptying of the bladder is a voluntary action.

The faecal waste fills the rectum and anal canal after absorption of the leftover water and salts by the large intestine. At this point of time, the nerves ending at the rectal region send a stimulus to our brain. The anus has internal involuntary and external voluntary anal sphincters. Our body then responds to the messages from the brain and voluntarily evicts the faecal waste at the appropriate time and place.

What happens inside a toddler who is not yet potty-trained:

The stimulus which are originated by the bladder reach up to the level of the spinal cord only and through a reflex bounce back. The child then poops as and when it receives the response. Here, no voluntary action is initiated by the child.

Voluntary responses start appearing at a later stage of growth of the child, which generally happens around the age of 2, sometimes a little earlier. However, this age varies from one child to another. Everybody is different. For some kids it can happen after 3-year-old. This is fine. If you are concerned about the time it takes for your child to reach that stage do not hesitate to speak to your pediatrician.

Classic Parents' Mistakes

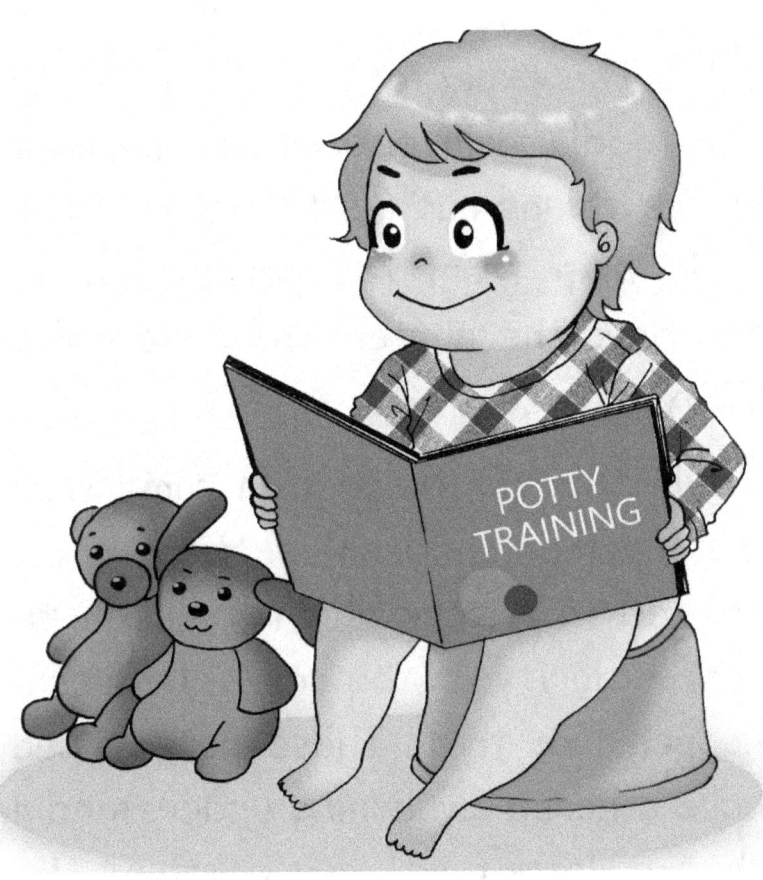

Potty-training? That's easy!

Many parents believe that since potty-training is a natural process, it will not take much effort, either on their part or on the part of their child. The expectation is that one day the toddler will be mature enough to figure things out (with, maybe, just a little help from the parents) and a few days thereafter, the child will be potty trained.

While this can be true in some cases with some children getting potty-trained in a very short time, in the vast majority of the cases, it doesn't happen like that. These parents may have a harsh awakening understanding that it is not as easy as they first thought. The disappointment can then turn into irritation and frustration.

No judgment here, just a reality. We're all humans. In turn, the parents' disappointment can reflect on the child's response making the process more difficult than it should be.

When young children have older brothers and sisters, things can be a little easier. They often show interest and curiosity for what their siblings do, and they usually want to know what happens in the bathroom. With these kids you have a better likelihood that they will understand by themselves what they should do after studying what their elders do. Often, they will even ask to follow them to the toilets.

A common misconception of Parents:

Parents usually look for general growth milestones and tend to base their expectations regarding toilet training age, temperament, readiness etc. on such milestones.

Readiness to potty-training bears no necessary relation to the achievements of these other growth milestones. They can be taken into account to gauge the readiness of the child to potty-train but various other factors, which we will discuss at a later stage of this book, also come into play.

Reliance on the advices of peers:

Many first-time parents, and sometimes parents with older children when faced with potty-training difficulties, try to gather information and advice from others, like relatives or friends.

The advice is most of the time provided based on the relatives or friends' own experience as to what worked well with their own kids. However, what the parents, and their friends or relatives, fail to realize is that at what age a child gets trained, how long the training takes or how smoothly it goes, varies from one child to another.

Previous success in potty-training:

Continuous dry days are usually taken as a conclusive evidence of success by most parents and they are taken aback when suddenly, the child experiences potty accidents. When this happens, the parents' expectations that they have succeeded in potty-training their child takes a hit and this can lead to frustrations. Some parents then show their unhappiness in front of the child which can make the situation.

Pushing for Early-Age Potty-Training:

Many parents have unrealistic expectations regarding the age at which their child should be potty trained. They also feel that the earlier the better and easier it will be for the child. Some feel pride in such a success, viewing it as indicator of how smart their child is.

While it is true that there are some parents who can potty-train their child successfully at a very early age, many others will not be able to reach this result right away. This can be frustrating and (which it might), may also put unnecessary expectations on the child, leading to unpleasant and unhealthy consequences such as regression.

The Readiness of The Child

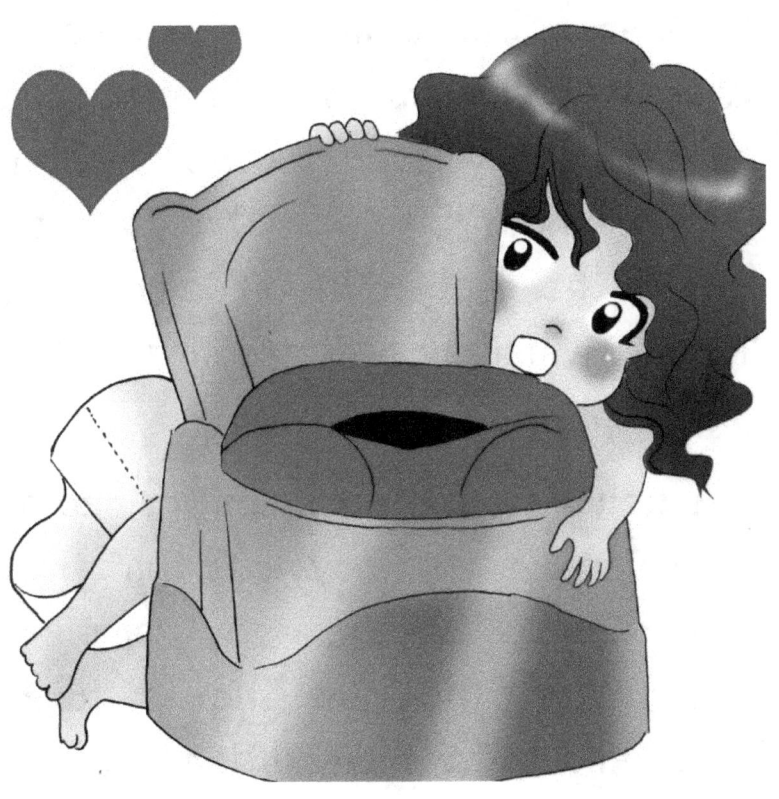

According to the American Academy of Pediatrics a child is ready to get potty-trained between the age of 18 months and 36 months. Again, the age is not set in stone and it differs from child to child. In recent years studies have shown that children now tend to be potty trained at a more advanced age than they used to be both in America and in Europe. This could be due to the availability of disposable diapers, which have made life easier for the parents.

It is believed that girls are trained at an earlier age than boys and that they take also lesser time to complete training. But the time that it takes for a child to be trained depends also from one child to another. While some children get trained in just a week or even less, others can take several months.

But let's be clear about what we mean by "being potty-trained". The standards may differ from one country to another but in North America and in Europe, "being potty trained" usually refers to the ability to go to the potty or toilet on time without making a mess but also to perform related actions such as the ability to go to the bathroom in the proper place and in the proper manner, to undress, to close bathroom doors, to properly wipe and flush the toilet paper, to dress again, etc.

Successful potty-training, rest assured, does not include night-time potty-training because most children may take a few more months or even years to become dry at night.

Indicators that your child is ready:

Toilet training should be started based on the physical abilities and mental maturity exhibited by the child. This will ensure that the child is physiologically and neurologically ready for performing independent toilet activities.

There are various ways a child will exhibit his or her readiness for potty-training. The signs to look for can be as follow:

- The child watches the toilet activities of others with interest;

- The child can walk and sit at one place continuously for at least some time, under guidance or following instructions;

- The child tries to imitate the actions of the peers;

- The child can retain fluid in, for a comparatively long time; say, about 2 hours or more;

- The child tries to pull off his pants and undergarments when feeling the urge to poop or pee;

- The child makes squirming or squatting or other typical actions when feeling the urge to poop or pee;

- The child can feel and express (in his own way), the inconvenience of having wet or soiled pants;

- The child tries to make signs that he would like to go to the toilets;

- The child has sufficient dexterity to pull up and down his pants and undergarments;

- Finally, the child satisfies certain psychological criteria like understanding simple verbal instructions and following them, so that the child is able to effectively carry out the necessary tasks associated with going to the bathroom.

These points are only a few and they are in no way exhaustive. Each child has its own way of expressing their readiness for potty training. Each toddler may show a few or most of the above pointers. It is your job as a parent to determine whether the time is right to start potty training them at that point, or to wait a little longer.

How Do Parents Go About Training Children?

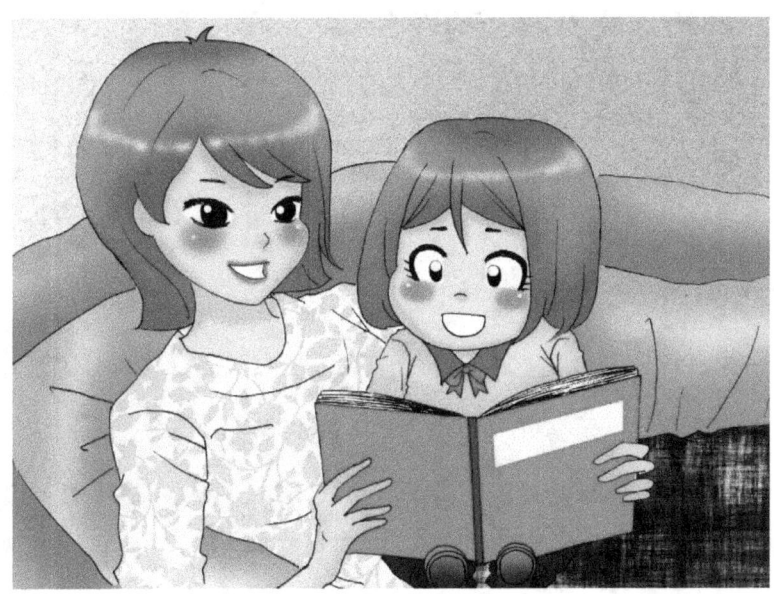

In practice, most parents start the potty-training process at the appropriate age (most often between 18/20 months old up to 2 to 2 ½ years old) after observing their child, or after being advised by their friends and very often by the grand-parents. In the vast majority of cases, the child successfully completes potty training quickly and continues with a problem-free childhood.

Outside North America and Europe, parents are well-known to start toilet training of their children at a much earlier age. This is possible in these countries because of the close physical proximity between parents and children round the clock, which helps parents predict when the child needs to go to the bathroom. Parents start training the child by taking it to the toilet to complete the activity. A point to be noted is that this purely entails avoidance at the specific place provided and does not include other activities like undressing, dressing, flushing, cleaning themselves etc. because the infant is usually not mature enough at this age to perform these activities.

The cases mentioned above describe ideal situations and while many parents and children are lucky enough to experience a smooth transition, others struggle with difficulties before transitioning.

In the subsequent chapters, we will discuss the difficulties faced in this regard, why such difficulties are encountered, and how they can be solved.

Main Potty-Training Methods

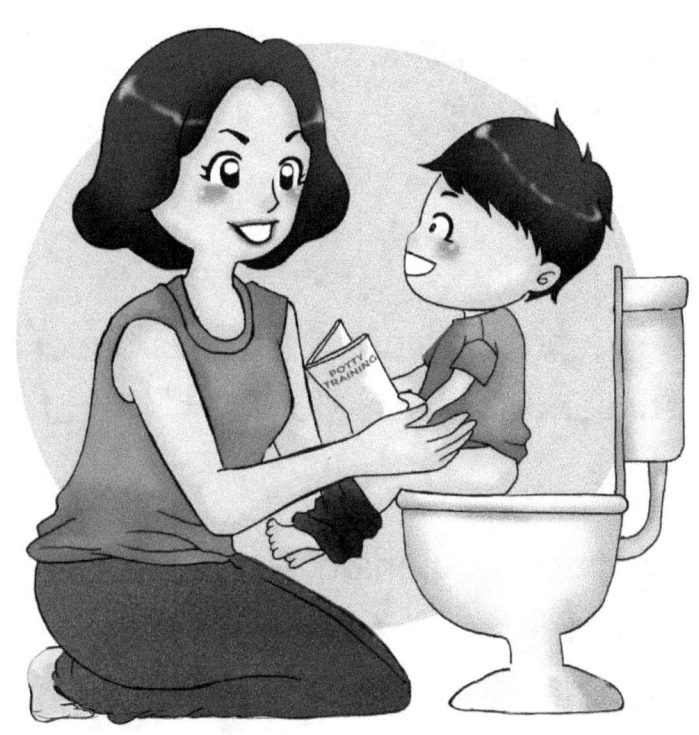

Potty Training in One Day

While getting children "potty-trained in a day" may sound far-fetched and impractical, experience shows otherwise. If not in a single day, within a few days, a child can get fully potty-trained.

Here is how it works:

- The potty training starts generally around 2-year-old (but it can be later);

- Before beginning the training, the child is taught all aspects of toilet training;

- Usually, a favourite superhero or doll is taken as an example and the parent teaches all the motions to be undertaken by the child through the doll. Because of the affinity of the child with the toy or with the doll, the instructions imparted via the toy or doll create a positive impression on the child;

- Parents can also give the doll or toy an incentive or a party when the doll successfully completes the potty training and performs all the associated activities;

- After the toddler comprehends fully what is expected, it is time to put the method into practice by the child himself. At this point, the child is mentally fully prepared to embark on the journey;

- The child wears training pants which gives a sense of encouragement and achievement;

- The little boy or the little girl is also given an encouragement in the form of an incentive or a party just like what was done with the toy or with the doll;

- An integral part of this method consists in giving the child something to drink when the child is thirsty. When the child feels the urge to go to the bathroom offer the child the possibility to use the bathroom. The child will use the potty which reduces the chances of 'accidents'. Of course, the child should not drink too much either, parents should remain reasonable!

The Conventional Method:

The most popular - and most successful – method is the following:

- The training can start around 2 years old ;

- The physiological, psychological and neurological development of the child are assessed by the parents to decide whether the child is ready for toilet training;

- The parents also assess whether the child can perform other tasks associated with our potty-training standards described above;

- The grandparents play a very important role in evaluating the readiness of the child, physically and emotionally, and the mindset of the parents etc;

- The parents remind the child when the child is expected to use the bathroom and gradually the child learns to intimate the parents when the need arises;

- An important aspect of this method is that the parents must praise the child for the successful attempts;

- Weaning the child away from diapers also plays a major role in giving confidence to the child;

- Caregivers should be kept informed of the developments and follow the method;

- This method also works for night-time training but it will usually take more time to work than for day-time training.

Assisted toilet training:

This method is also sometimes called the "elimination communication" method or "EC" method. It is used in a number of countries and is known to be a popular method in China. This method requires a very close proximity of at least one of the parents with the child. The training usually starts somewhere around the age of 6 months and involves the absence of diapers. Yes, you read it correctly, no diaper.

As its name suggests this method is based on communication between the parent and the child. The parent must look for the signals that the child needs to go. The parent will then bring the child to the potty or to the toilets and will hold him over the potty.

The parent should also keep track of the usual time the child needs to go and offers the child to the possibility to go by bringing the child and holding him over the potty.

At the time of going to the bathroom, the parent should make a distinctive sound, which sounds will then be associated in the child's mind with going to the potty. This sound will later be used to indicate that the child must go the potty.

Although this method is prevalent in some places, because of the practical difficulties (necessity to be close at all time) it may be a little challenging to follow by parents who both work. It is still possible however to use it when with the child but, in this case, it will have to be associated with diapers to avoid too many accidents.

Problems Faced by Parents

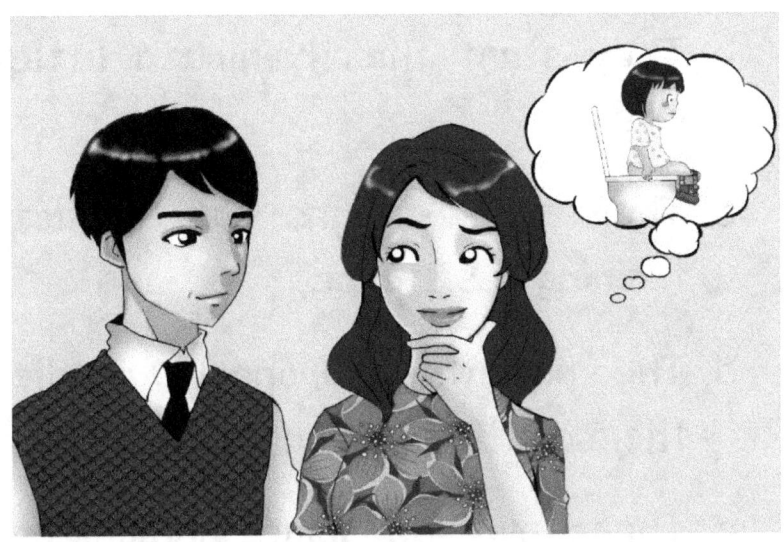

In practice, many children face certain difficulties, mainly because of the following reasons:

a. They start toilet training at an early age

b. They start the training a little late

c. They show signs of "toilet training resistance"

d. The parents improperly handle them at the training stage

e. There may be some medical or physical reasons.

Let's look at each of these reasons one after the other.

Toilet-training at an early age

Early toilet training may lead to day-wetting and constipation. Unrestricted voidance in the diaper by young children who are not ready for toilet training is usually considered beneficial for the normal growth and expansion of the bladder. If, on the other hand, they start training before their bodies are ready, the children may tend to hold back urine and stools for longer periods which is detrimental to bladder growth. According to a research conducted by the Wake Forest Baptist Medical Center starting potty training too early, before the age of 2, could cause daytime wetting problems at a later stage. Also, because the stool is retained for longer periods, these children are prone to constipation.

Besides, it may lead to frustrations, negative attitude and other psychological repercussions.

Hence, it is wiser not to pressure a child into the potty-training process before the child is ready to handle it. This is something that parents can and should discuss with their pediatrician.

Starting potty-training late

Delaying training to a later age (past 36 months) can also be equally detrimental according to the same study mentioned above and cited at the end this book. It could lead to problems like constipation. In addition, the child may also refuse to go to the bathroom since the child wasn't trained in due time.

Children showing "toilet training resistance"

Some children, who seem to be physically and physiologically ready to be potty-trained, categorically refuse all of their parents' attempts to train them.

If a child of 3 years of age or more, whom the parents have been trying to train for quite some time, refuses to use the potty or toilets for unknown reasons, then such

child can be considered as a child who is training-resistant.

There are children, who, even if placed over the potty or a toilet, will not go and they will prefer to soil their diapers *right after* getting off the potty!! This can be very frustrating for parents. Other children, instead, end up soiling themselves, holding back on bowel movement, leading to constipation.

There may be many various reasons explaining this kind of behaviour. The child may be stubborn, strong-willed, disinterested or simply afraid of the toilet. In some cases, the resistance exhibited may even be a form of revolt against parental insistence.

So, what can the parents do to overcome this situation?

- *Stop* reminding the child to use the potty. These children do not want to follow the (direct) instructions of their parents, so a strategy can consist in indirectly encouraging the child to use the toilet to give the child a sense of achieving success *on his own.* It works wonders.

- Since the child is already mature enough to understand most oral instructions, the parents should *make it clear that using the potty, not soiling underpants and maintaining cleanliness by disposing of the waste at the* *proper place **is the child's own responsibility.***

- Stop using diapers and training pants or use them less. It will push the child to visit the toilets when needed because at this age the child will be mature enough to understand that soiled underwear is not comfortable.

- When a child not only refuses to use the toilets but also tries to stop the urge for bowel movements, it might **lead to constipation** and to other medical problems. To avoid this, parents should sit with the child and explain to their son or daughter why it's a good thing to eliminate. There are many books and DVDs designed to explain the potty-training process to a very young audience. Parents can use one of these books or video programs as an educational tool.

- Choose a toy, a game, a doll or even a cartoon that the child truly likes and use them as an incentive when the child uses the potty properly. The allowance is for a limited time only and under the control of the parent so that the child appreciates the **importance of the incentive.**

- Make it a point to document the achievements on a chart and show the same to the family physician at the time of visit and praise the child for the improvement. A praise or encouragement in the presence of an authority figure such as the family physician gives good impetus to the child to stick to good habits.

- Some children might resist potty training due to phobias. It's a classic. Some children are afraid that they may fall into the toilet. In such a case, it would be advisable to use a small stool or a box to sit the child more comfortably and to feel confident. If you use a box, make sure that it is safe and that the child cannot fall from it when leaving the toilets and fall into it. Alternately, a potty can be used until such time that the child starts feeling confident enough to use the toilets. Conversely, if the child does not like a potty, the parents can encourage the child to directly use the toilet at home. The comfort of the child is really important.

Improper handling of the children by the parents

Whatever method the parents want to adopt to potty-train their child, there are certain things **to do** and certain things that should **not to be done** if they want a smooth transition.

Some things to do:

a. Pay close attention to the maturity of your child and to the various milestones achieved to decide if this is the right time and *then* start potty-training. This can be discussed with your pediatrician. You do not necessarily have to make that decision on your own.

- This happens to be ***the most*** important step in toilet training a child since many aspects of mental maturation, physical readiness, willingness etc. contribute to success or failure of the toilet training exercise.

b. Choose a potty that the child likes or let the child use the toilet if this is its choice. Make the potty or toilet a pleasant place to be because the child should feel comfortable and stress-free when visiting it.

c. Choose the time the child is likely to use the potty and lead it to the potty. This is only a temporary phase. The ultimate goal is to get the child to go to the toilet by himself.

d. The transition from wearing diapers to training pants should be explained to the child by putting this into perspective. Of course, we are talking about a young child but with the proper words this can be easily achieved. The idea it to make him understand the importance of the leap he is making, which in turn, will encourage him to take pride in the achievement instead of treating it as a compulsory hurdle to be crossed.

e. Praises and incentives must be a part of the training process to make it a pleasurable journey for the child.

What are the "No No's"?

a. **The first, and the most important of all, is that you should *not compel the child to train*,** under any circumstances. It could foster rebellion and ultimately make things more complicated than they should be.

b. Accidents and regression *after* the toilet training is completed are quite common. The parents should **not show their disappointment or frustration** because it could reflect on the child's behaviour.

c. Some children will not adjust easily and smoothly to toilet training. They may also take a long time to train, much to the frustration of the parents. Again, **at no time should the child witness your frustration.**

d. The child should ***never be punished*** for lack of improvement, resistance, accidents, regression, etc.

e. Do not make the child sit on the potty for a long stretch of time, waiting that whatever should

55

happen happens. This will likely result in rebellion.

f. **Do not restrict the child's physical activities** as a method of punishment because it will, in fact, have an adverse impact on proper avoidance. Physical activity helps in maintaining your child's good health and well-being, which is a key factor in good bowel movement.

Medical Problems

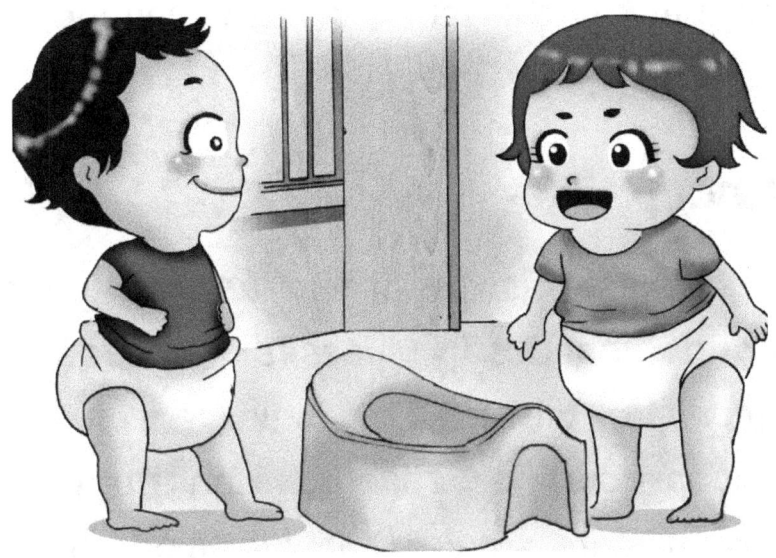

In some cases, medical problems can interfere with the potty-training. These should always be brought to the attention of your pediatrician. Two conditions in particular can play a role in the difficulty of the training.

Encopresis

Encopresis is the term used when a child repeatedly passes faeces at improper places. The main reason for encopresis is chronic constipation, which can come from stress, from fiber deficiency, from the fact that the child does not drink enough water, or from some medical reason such as a sore near the anus etc.

This should be discussed with your pediatrician and one of the solutions usually involves a diet or a change in toilet habits to enable the child to pass stools easily and fully.

If the cause of the problem is the child's anxiety the parents will need to provide a stress-free atmosphere and environment. In some cases, psychotherapy may also be recommended.

Enuresis

Enuresis is a form of incontinence. Basically, the child cannot control when he pees. Most of the time, problems happen during bed time, but, the child may also have daytime wetting accidents. Neither daytime nor bedtime wetting are voluntary for the child, and hence it should be made very clear to the child that he should not feel guilty because it is not the child's fault.

When Should the Parents Seek Help?

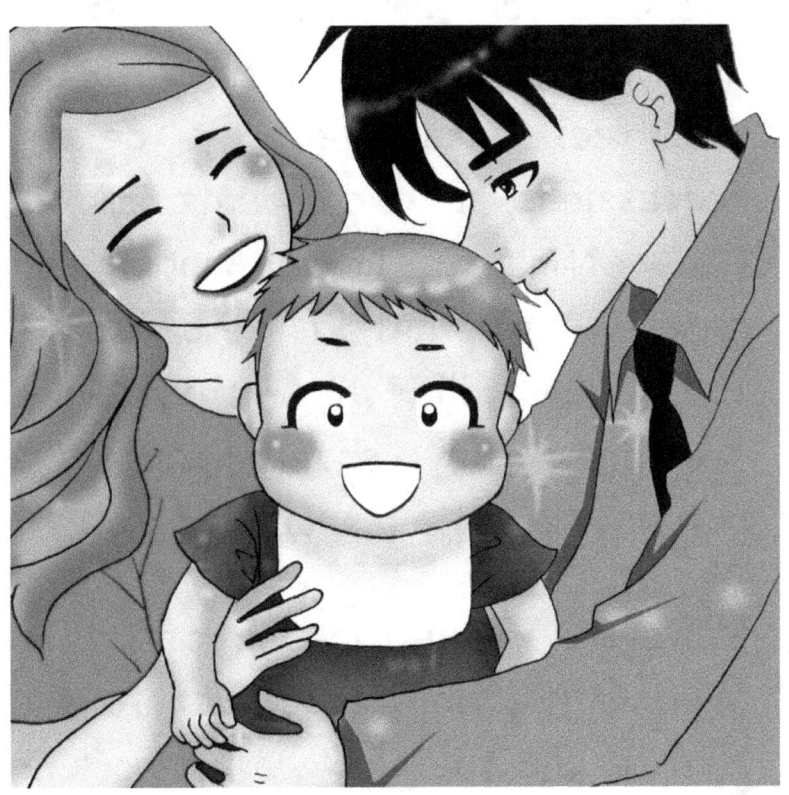

As we said, how long it takes to become potty-trained is going to depend on many different factors. It can take very little time, or it can take more efforts. Because it takes more time than the parents imagine it should does not mean that there is anything wrong. Parents should not feel frustrated by delays, regressions, potty accidents or even bed-wetting etc. It can happen, and chances are that it happened to them as well when they were toddlers. They should persevere patiently to obtain positive results.

However, if by the age of 3 the child is not able to adjust to the routine and they have been working on it for quite some time, or it appears that the child might have some medical problem like constipation or diarrhea, they *should* consider obtaining expert advice.

Potty-training is also a question that can be raised any time the parents bring their child to the doctor, even if it's for a routine visit or at the occasion of vaccinations and normal check-ups. What many parents ignore is that often they can just call their doctor and discuss the issue, or any other issues they may be experiencing, over the phone rather than going to visit the doctor's office, which may sometimes be difficult when both parents are working.

64

Children With Special Needs

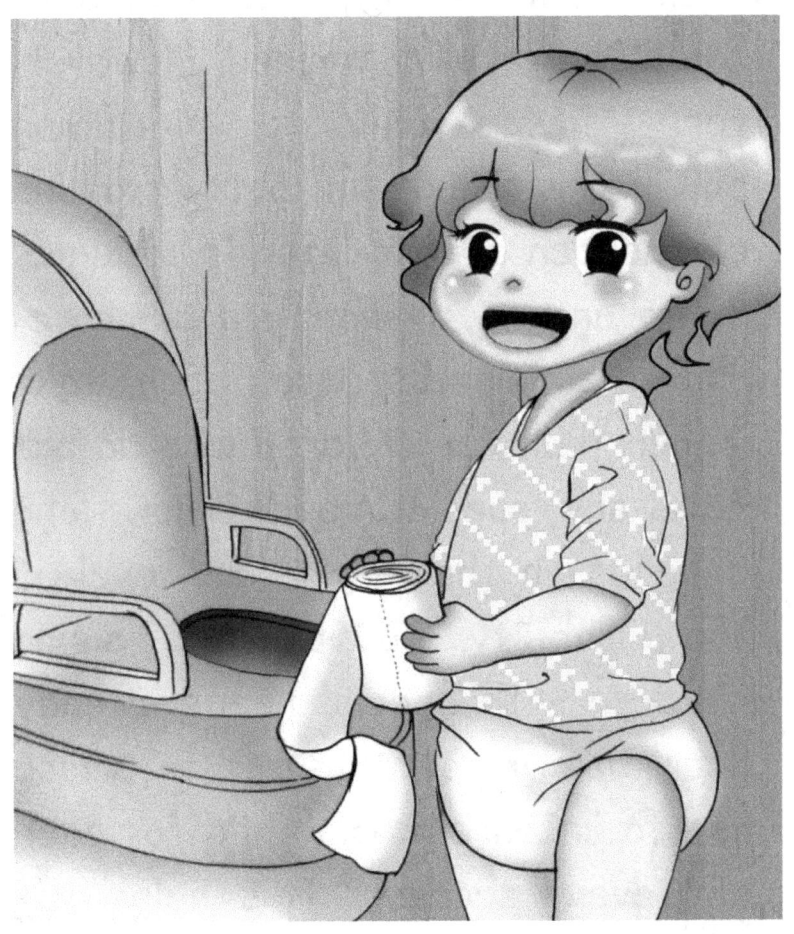

Potty-training children with special needs can sometimes seem more challenging. Parents should not be disheartened. With the help of their pediatrician, these children can also be potty-trained. However, for these children, including children with autism, potty-training can happen a little later (sometimes up to around 5 years-old or more) and the process itself can take longer than for children who do not have any special needs. How long depends on the nature and level of the disability. But parents raising children with special needs already know how important it is to praise and to encourage the child for each and every success. This helps the child gain a sense of achievement.

In a nutshell, parents of special needs children should anticipate that the potty-training process will take longer than what they might expect, and they should address the question with their doctor to see what would be the best approach based on the specific needs of the child.

Some Final Tips

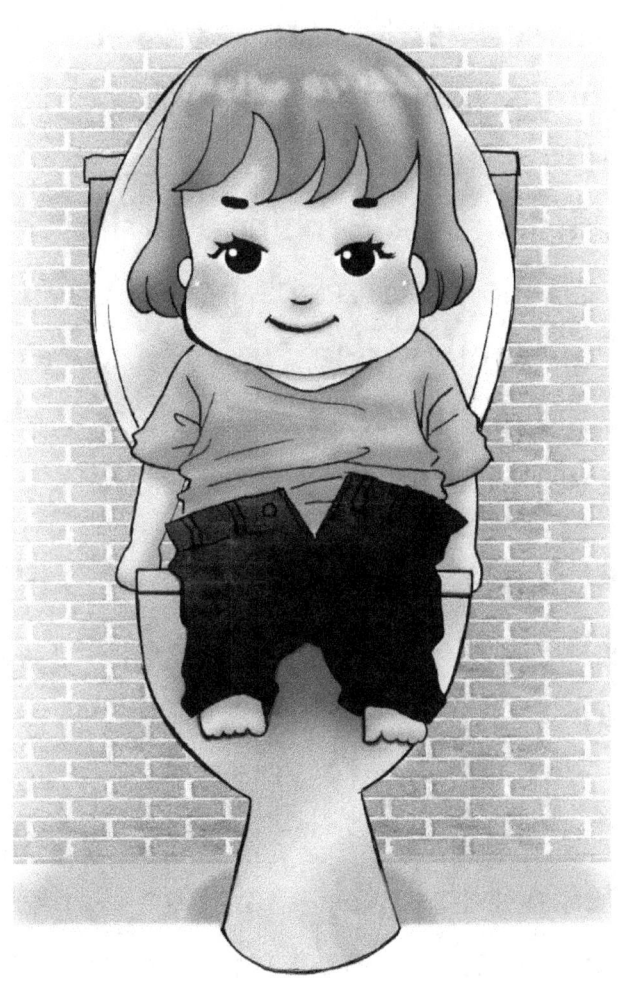

- Do not compare your child with others. Each child is different, and many factors come into play: age, temperament, family environment, gender... A lot of things count when it comes to potty-training successes. **All children** get trained ultimately; a few months/years earlier or later. This milestone is in no way a barometer or a sign of the child's level intelligence.

- At least 3 to 5 percent of children go through some hiccups before they can become fully potty-trained, due to various reasons. It could be due to their different temperaments, minor medical reasons, or even for no reason at all! All it takes is patience and perseverance.

- Most of the time, parents are able to gauge the child's preparedness and instinctively find the correct method of 'how-to' and are able to achieve smooth success. When in doubt, never hesitate to seek guidance of the family pediatrician.

- Parents of children with special needs should seek the assistance of an expert (i.e. a doctor!) at every step of the way. These children also need a lot of attention, care and sensitivity.

- Never, ever, get irritated with the child for accidents, regressions or for any other problem. It can only aggravate the problem and make things more complicated.

- Last but not the least, all it needs is a lot of encouragement, praise, some incentives, lots of love on the part of the parent, and both the parent and the child will come out with flying colours!

Conclusion

Potty-training is an important milestone of your child's development. If you are lucky enough your child will pass with flying colours. If a little less fortunate, give your child some time and do not pressure him too much or this could end up having the exact opposite result than the one you expected. Never show anger or frustration. It's never fun to have to deal with pee on the carpet or soiled clothes to wash, let's face it, but it's not intentional, it's not again you and it's in no way intended to make your life more difficult. It's simply part of a natural process and your child will eventually be successful.

Potty-training should not start too early or too late either. Look for signs of readiness. Follow the potty-training method that's best suited for the child, keep the child healthy with a proper diet, and well hydrated, show patience and the job will be done. Smoothly and painlessly, for all concerned.

I hope you enjoyed this book and found it useful. If so, please do not hesitate to leave a review! It really helps!

References

Articles

Stadtler AC, Gorski PA, Brazelton TB. Toilet Training Methods, Clinical Interventions, and Recommendations. American Academy of Pediatrics. Pediatrics 1999; 103:1359.

Martin JA, King DR, Maccoby EE, and Jaklin CN. 1984. Secular Trends and Individual Differences in Toilet-Training Progress. Journal of Pediatric Psychology 9: 457-468.

Largo RH, Molinari L, von Siebenthal K, and Wolfensberger U. 1996. Does a profound change in toilet-training affect development of bowel and bladder control? Dev Med Child Neurol. 38:1106-16.

Bakker E; Wyndaele JJ. 2000. Changes in the toilet training of children during the last 60 years: the cause of an increase in lower urinary tract dysfunction? British journal of Urology, 86(3):248-52.

Hodges, S. J., Richards, K. A., Gorbachinsky, I., & Krane, L. S. (2014). The association of age of toilet training and dysfunctional voiding. *Research and Reports in Urology*, *6*, 127-130.

http://doi.org/10.2147/RRU.S66839

Brazelton TB (1962) A child-oriented approach to toilet training. Pediatrics. 29:121–128.

Books

Diaper Free! The Gentle Wisdom of Natural Infant Hygiene. Natural Wisdom Press (2001) Ingrid Bauer.

Toilet Training in Less Than a Day. Pocket Books (1989) Azrin Nathan H, Foxx Richard M.

Little People: Guidelines for Commonsense Child Rearing. 4th ed. Overland Press Inc (1988) Christophersen Edward R.

Other Publication

American Academy of Pediatrics. *Toilet Training. Guidelines for Parents.* Elk Grove Village, Il: AAP; 1998.

Websites

https://www.aap.org

https://www.wakehealth.edu/News-Releases/2014/Potty_Training_Before_Age_2_Linked_to_Increased_Risk_of_Later_Wetting_Problems,_Research_Shows.htm

www.ingramcontent.com/pod-product-compliance
Lightning Source LLC
Chambersburg PA
CBHW052335220526
45472CB00001B/441